How to age positively

A handbook for personal change in later life

Acknowledgments

Various colleagues have helped me develop my thinking around positive ageing. Worthy of special mention are Dave Griffiths, with whom I started on the journey, and John Drowley and Julie Cooke who also joined in. I am indebted to my wife Ruth Holland who has supported me throughout and who first of all brought my attention to the work of Marie de Hennezel who stimulated a huge amount of my interest in this area. I would also like to thank Pip Morgan for his excellent work in editing my original manuscript.

"Something within us does not grow old. I shall call it the heart. I don't mean the organ, which does of course age, but the capacity to love and desire. The heart I refer to is that inexplicable, incomprehensible force which keeps the human being alive... It is this heart that can help us to push on through our fears, and bear us up amid the worst ordeals of old age."

Marie de Hennezel, from *The warmth of the heart prevents your body from rusting: Ageing without growing old* [1]

How to age positively: a handbook for personal change in later life.

Published by Positive Ageing Associates, Bristol
All Rights Reserved ©Positive Ageing Associates

First published in 2014

Interior and cover design by In The Dog House Design
www.bazziel.wix.com/inthedoghousedesign

Printed and bound by Lightning Source UK Ltd

ISBN: 978-0-9930559-0-4

Positive Ageing
Associates

www. positiveageingassociates.com

Contents

INTRODUCTION

The prospect for people over 60 has never looked so promising as it does now! Men and women at retirement age can expect to live for a further 20 years on average, and for most of that time they are likely to be in good health. But it's not just a matter of living longer: the over-60s can actually look forward to a whole new phase in life – a period that could be longer than all the time they spent at school!

This new phase is filled with great potential, with plenty of opportunities for learning, engaging in new activities, travelling, giving back to society, being creative etc. We can make the best of this time if we approach it with a positive mental attitude and make some simple preparations. **How to age positively: a handbook for personal change in later life** offers a route map to help people find their way through the changes they face and a toolkit of exercises to help them reach their chosen path and fulfil their potential.

This book on ageing is probably unlike any other you have read. We don't look at things such as exercise or diet (although these are important), but concentrate instead on the purely psychological and emotional aspects of ageing. Moreover, we provide a wealth of scientific evidence – and many specific references – to back up and sustain our views on the benefits of positive ageing.

The problem with ageing arises from fears and misunderstandings, which ultimately lead so many people to avoid thinking about it altogether. However, like most things in life, "burying your head in the sand" is not very helpful. Much better to face the issue head on – and this book is designed to help you do precisely that.

Just as we had to learn to grow up, so we have to learn to grow old. If we don't put some thought and attention into preparing for these years then we could very easily feel short-changed or disappointed. However, if we take some time to look closely at the issues, we are much more likely to age well and reap the benefits.

WHAT IS AGE AND AGEING?

Surprisingly, there is no simple answer to the question – "What is ageing"! It can be very misleading to think of age and ageing as simply a chronological progression of the number of years a person has lived. Someone who is 60 can look and behave like a 40-year-old, and another person who is 40 can look and feel like a 60 year old. So it is much more complicated than a simple numbers game.

There are three main ways of understanding ageing:

Biological – ageing brings physical changes in the body; most obviously wrinkles and grey hair. But these can give a misleading or partial view because some people can get wrinkles and grey hair much younger or older than others. Not only is it impossible to tell someone's age from any particular physical feature or specific internal process, but there is no medical test to determine how old someone is. As one of the country's leading experts, Professor Tom Kirkwood, says – *"Ageing appears to be a lifelong accumulation of faults at the cellular and molecular level, each a random occurrence insignificant in itself, combining to overwhelm the body's ability to keep its systems running. The random nature of these faults is what makes us each age so individually, and it is this individuality and the underlying complexity, which makes the ageing process such an intriguing scientific challenge."*

Psychological – ageing is also commonly associated with changes in personality and mental states. Most obviously there are stereotypes about older people being forgetful and grumpy. In reality these ideas owe more to ageism than science. There is no research evidence that links later life with becoming grumpy or loss of significant mental functioning.

Cultural – society has a big part to play in how we define age. For example, an older person is commonly thought of as 'a pensioner', but when this is, depends on current legislation because the state pension age changes. (It is interesting to note that when pensions were first introduced the age of entitlement was 70!). Culture can determine our sense of how old we are – for example, ideas such as "60 is the new 40". We are also influenced by media images of older people: on one extreme, the frail and rather miserable older person and on the other extreme, the 'superhero' 100 year old marathon runner. Neither is truly representative: we need more mature and varied images in the media.

So there is no simple or objective way of defining age and ageing. Perhaps we should rely on a much more subjective view of age and ageing. It may really be best to stick with that old adage that 'you are only as old as you feel'.

WHAT IS POSITIVE AGEING?

Let's start with what it is not! In our view of the world, positive ageing is not about fighting against or denying the ageing process, or trying to live extraordinary lengths of time, with no wrinkles! Nor is it about amassing a large fortune. The answer is much more meaningful and complex.

What would it mean to age well or successfully? A great deal of academic thinking and research has been spent on trying to find answers to this question.

One of the classic academic definitions of successful ageing [2] is:

• an absence of disease
• the maintenance of physical and mental functioning
• an active and independent engagement with life

This is a helpful definition, but it is incomplete because it misses a number of important things. In her detailed study of the literature around 'successful ageing[3] Professor Ann Bowling sets out (see list below) the elements from three main viewpoints – biomedical, psychosocial and the general public perspective (noting that there was some overlap).

Main elements of successful ageing:-

• Greater life expectancy
• Improving life satisfaction and wellbeing
• Having good mental and psychological health and cognitive function

- Achieving personal growth, including learning new things
- Maintaining good physical health and functioning
- Psychological characteristics including a sense of autonomy, control, independence, adaptability, coping, self-esteem, positive outlook, and positive sense of self
- Access to leisure activities and participation in the local community
- Participation in satisfying social networks
- Accomplishing several goal
- Achieving financial security
- Living in a desirable neighbourhood
- Having a sense of contributing to life
- Displaying a sense of humour
- Gaining a sense of purpose
- Developing one's spirituality

Shorter summaries of ageing well can also be helpful. For example, some researchers [4] think that people will find wellbeing in later life when they achieve the following six aspects of wellness:

- **Self-Acceptance** – positive thinking about oneself and one's past life
- **Personal Growth** – a sense of continued growth and development as a person
- **Purpose in Life** – belief that one's life is purposeful and meaningful
- **Positive Relations With Others** – the possession of quality relations with others
- **Environmental Mastery** – the capacity to manage effectively one's life and surrounding world
- **Autonomy** – a sense of self-determination.

This search for the key elements of successful ageing may seem rather academic, but it is important. Most discussion tends to concentrate solely on the biological components of physical health. In other words, the thinking tends to be very medically focused. However, when older people themselves are asked for their definition of successful ageing, whilst physical health is their most important factor, the next most important elements are more to do with feelings and friendships with others[3] . These include:

- A positive outlook and self worth
- A sense of control over life
- Independence
- Effective coping strategies to help deal with life's changing challenges
- Social role and activities.

See opposite page for a pragmatic distillation of the various academic modelling of the components for successful ageing.

Let's look at each of these 'branches' of successful ageing in turn:

PHYSICAL HEALTH

In very simple terms – and leaving aside certain genetic factors – a person can significantly enhance and maintain their physical health through a good diet and regular exercise. [The public health messages are very prevalent, and the issues and requirements are well documented with a huge wealth of reference material available. That is why there is no need for us to go into any detail here.]

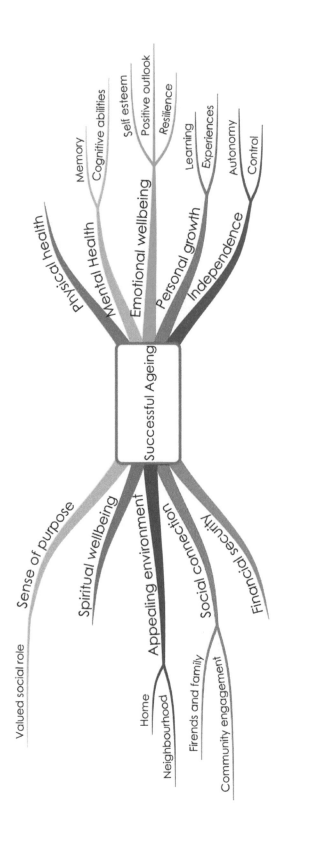

Source: Guy Robertson

MENTAL HEALTH

The old saying that *'there is a sound mind in a healthy body'* holds much truth. Our mental health can be significantly influenced by our physical health and vice versa. Many people are very worried about losing their thinking skills when they get older, yet the research is much more positive than the general public's ideas on ageing. For example, our general knowledge as well as our vocabulary and learned skills, including some number skills, often stay pretty well intact, even into very old age[5] . What's more, there are activities to help people retain their memory and cognitive abilities. Although the scientific studies are not conclusive about whether 'brain training' works, it is nevertheless clear that people who engage in mental activities have a richer mental life[5]. Those wishing to pursue this further could look at Tony Buzan's book *Age-proof Your Brain*.

EMOTIONAL WELLBEING

Both physical and mental health have an impact on emotional wellbeing, and vice versa. As we will learn later, emotional wellbeing and happiness generally increase with age. The key elements to pay attention to are:

- **Self esteem** – feeling good about oneself
- **Optimistic outlook** – having a positive framework makes a very real difference
- **Resilience** – having a mental attitude that allows one to bounce back from the crises and challenges that hit us from time to time. It's not what happens to you in life that's important, it's how you respond to it.

PERSONAL GROWTH

Continuing to develop oneself by engaging fully in life's rich array of experiences and opportunities for learning is very important in later years. Older people need to believe that there's no end to learning and that they need to sustain this belief.

INDEPENDENCE

One of the biggest fears that people have about ageing is the potential loss of autonomy and control over their lives and living situations. But contrary to the general public's perception, illness and disability do not necessarily need to compromise them. There are many examples of people with severe impairments leading very active and independent lives.

FINANCIAL SECURITY

This is self-evident but very important. There is a huge amount of advice available on how to manage resources in later life so this issue is not addressed further in this book.

SOCIAL CONNECTION

Independence is important, but so is **interdependence**. Human beings are social animals and relationships with others and engagement in local communities is fundamental to their wellbeing. Indeed, research shows that loneliness is as harmful to wellbeing as smoking 15 cigarettes a day [6]. Not everyone needs the same level of interaction, but we all need to achieve the level that satisfies us and keeps us from feeling lonely.

APPEALING ENVIRONMENT

As we get older our homes and neighbourhoods tend to become more important to us. We are likely to spend more time in them than perhaps we did when we worked full time for example. Ensuring one's living situation is fit for later life is a crucial part of positive ageing.

SPIRITUAL WELLBEING

Impending death makes a difference to how one views the world and one's life. That is not to say that everyone becomes spiritual, but it does mean that making sense of life and the world can become more important. There are a variety of ways – guidelines, practices, etc – of achieving spiritual wellbeing, including through philosophical understanding or the resolution of old existential questions.

SENSE OF PURPOSE

A sense of purpose is one of the most beneficial things for our health and wellbeing in later life. People who know what their purpose in life is live longer and better lives[7]. It can be a challenge to establish ones sense of purpose in later life – particularly if full time employment previously provided a lot of meaning.

IN SUMMARY

Successful ageing is most likely to be achieved where people take some care over their body, mind, emotional wellbeing and social life. Given the prevalence of ageist attitudes towards later life it is particularly important that people consciously root out negative attitudes towards ageing and replace them with a more positive perspective. It is this that is the key to developing a positive ageing perspective.

... the more we're able to understand how ageist assumptions shape our thoughts and behaviour, the less hold they will have over us... As we begin to identify the caricatures and prejudices we've internalised and understand their social origins, they become more resistable. And this makes it more possible to age more freely - to become more fully ourselves.

Anne Karpf [28]

EXPLODING
SOME
MYTHS

Most people tend to have very negative ideas about ageing. The reality however is usually very different. What follows is an outline of, and challenge to, four of the most common myths about ageing.

MYTH ONE:
AGEING IS A STEADY DOWNWARD SPIRAL

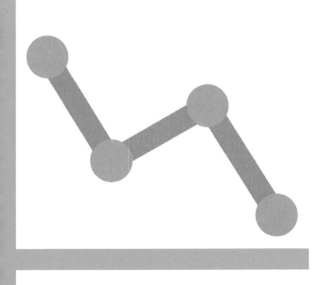

People often think that when they reach old age, they will either develop dementia or they will soon be so physically unwell that life won't be worth living.

The risk of developing an illness increases directly with age. This is clearly true but it is greatly exaggerated, although there are variations – for example, poorer people experience greater ill-health, and this should be borne in mind when considering the figures provided here.

For people over 65 in the UK:

● Around 60% report that no illness is limiting their lifestyle[8]

● Can expect to live in good health for around 60% of their remaining life (there are some slight differences between men and women), according to government statistics[8].

ASK THE 'OLDEST OLD'

Even when people do fall ill in later life, the experience is very different from what most people would believe. For example, a study of the 'oldest old' – people over 85 – found that, although everyone by that age had some form of health problem, only 20% of them required any professional care or support to enable them to live independently[9]. More importantly, nearly 80% of them rated their health and quality of life as "good, very good, or excellent"! So the lived experience of older people is very different from the stereotype of illness, disease and distress.

FIGURES ABOUT DEMENTIA

Even with dementia the reality is very different from what most people imagine, which is probably fuelled by press stories about 'an epidemic of Alzheimer's Disease' sweeping the country. The latest figures from the Alzheimer's Society paint a very different picture [10]. In the UK, 1 in 6 people over 80 (the most susceptible group) are likely to develop some form of dementia. There is no denying that this is a lot of people – but more importantly, it means that the overwhelming majority (about 84%) of people over 80 do not develop dementia. Only 1% of those aged 65 to 69 develop it. And there is even some evidence emerging to suggest that the incidence of dementia is declining[11].

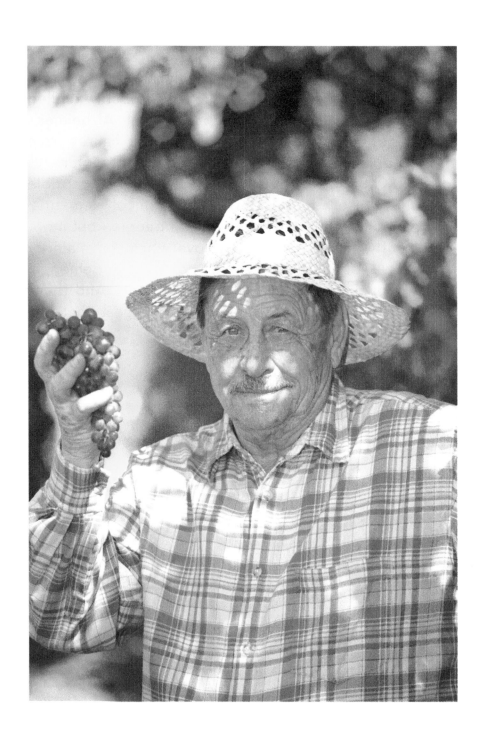

MYTH TWO:
OLD AGE IS A MISERABLE TIME

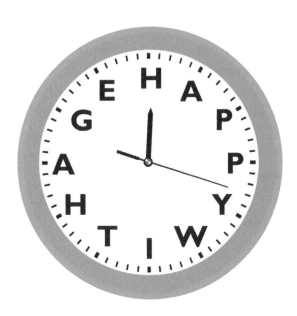

Nothing couldn't be further from the truth. Countless surveys have shown that, as people grow older, they generally get happier. In fact, the most unhappy people are those in mid-life (45-49). Life satisfaction is particularly high for older people between 65-79, with some tailing off for those over 80[12].

COMPARE YOUNG AND OLD

With the exception of dementia (see Myth One, page 15), emotional and mental health generally improves with age. Compared with younger people, older people suffer less from depression, anxiety and drug abuse. They tend to experience fewer negative emotions, and when these emotions do arise they tend to process or deal with them more quickly and have greater control over them [12, 13]. Emotional wellbeing therefore appears to improve with ageing, resulting in older people demonstrating greater emotional stability and reduced emotional intensity [14].

WHY SHOULD THIS BE?

Well according to Stanford psychologist Laura Carstensen it is explained by her 'socioemotional selectivity theory'[15]. In summary, this theory suggests that, as time horizons shrink, as they do with ageing, people become increasingly selective and invest more of their emotional resources in meaningful goals and activities. This in turn affects how people's mental attention and memory works. Older people develop a greater tendency to pay attention to and remember positive rather than negative information, images and events. And because they tend to place much more importance on emotional satisfaction, older people tend to spend more time with familiar friends with whom they have rewarding relationships. This maximizes the chance of positive emotional experiences.

MYTH THREE:
PHYSICAL ILLNESS IS COMPLETELY IS COMPLETELY BEYOND PEOPLE'S CONTROL

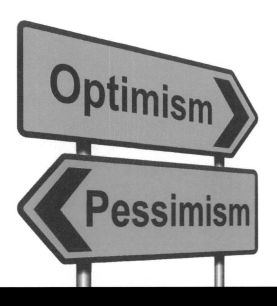

R esearch shows that our minds can have a very significant impact on our body and our physical health. In fact, an overwhelming amount of evidence reveals that happier people live longer. For example, a large review of more than 160 scientific studies found "clear and compelling evidence" that happy people tend to live longer and experience better health than their unhappy peers[16].

Here are some research results:

• One study found that people who are depressed or anxious are much more likely to have heart disease[17].

• Another study found that moods such as joy and happiness, as well as characteristics such as hopefulness, optimism and a sense of humour were associated with greater predicted longevity[18].

• In a large-scale study, nearly 5,000 students who filled out an optimism scale when they started university in 1964–66 were followed for 40 years. It found that pessimistic individuals died earlier than more optimistic students[19].

• A study of recovery rates from heart surgery found that recovery was quicker for optimists[20].

• A two year study of over 400 hip-fracture patients aged 65 and older showed that high positive emotional wellbeing was associated with faster walking and chair-stand speeds[21].

BENEFITS OF BEING OPTIMISTIC

So, overall, the research shows that optimism appears to have a number of health and wellbeing benefits:

• Increased life span

• Lower rates of depression

• Lower levels of distress

• Greater resistance to the common cold

• Better psychological and physical wellbeing

• Reduced risk of death from cardiovascular disease

• Better coping skills during hardships and times of stress.

Optimism has been shown to explain between 5-10% of the variation in the likelihood of developing some health conditions, including:

• Cardiovascular disease[20]

• Stroke[22]

• Depression[23]

• Cancer[24]

A large review of the evidence has confirmed that optimism is related to psychological wellbeing[25]. A quote from the study says: *"Put simply, optimists emerge from difficult circumstances with less distress than do pessimists."*

A quote from another study [25] says: *"Optimists seem intent on facing problems head-on, taking active and constructive steps to solve their problems; pessimists are more likely to abandon their effort to attain their goals."*

So how we think about and deal with our problems can make a real difference to how long and how well we live.

The general conclusion from all these studies is that feeling positive about life helps people to live longer and in better health. Optimism is therefore very important to our health and wellbeing, particularly as we get older.

MYTH FOUR:
HOW LONG PEOPLE LIVE IS DETERMINED BY THEIR GENES

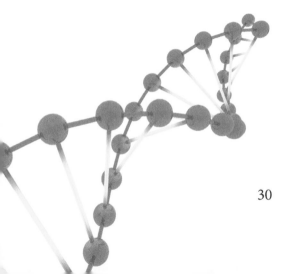

Many people think that their lifespan is some kind of family trait that is determined by their genes. For example, people often assume they will have the same sort of lifespan as their parents or grandparents. The reality is that there is no biological or genetic programme determining when we will die. Whilst there are some family trends in longevity, the contribution from our genes is only about a quarter of what determines our length of life[26].

Studies have shown quite clearly that the age of parents or grandparents isn't a very important predictor of individual lifespan. A quote from one study[27] says: *"Human beings do not have a single gene that controls age itself, or that programs when you'll die."*

Even where there is a genetic link to a specific medical condition, that genetic predisposition is not the same as a prediction. In other words, the medical condition will not occur in all cases.

WHAT TWINS REVEAL ABOUT AGEING

The evidence on this comes from numerous studies of twins. A quote from a study on twins[27] says: *"Twin studies have made it abundantly clear that even two people with the same birthday and parents – and in the case of identical twins, the exact same DNA – can have different health and ageing trajectories."* The study provides examples of twins, where one twin has exercised while the other has not, and where as a result, they live for different lengths and have different health outcomes.

So genes do have some influence, but they are not the determining factor.

Research suggests that people have much more control over how long and how well they live than they commonly think. The main message from research can be summarised by a quote from one study[2]:

"We can have a dramatic impact on our own success or failure in ageing. Far more than is usually assumed, successful ageing is in our own hands."

The wealth of evidence from research is very positive and shatters the myth that we have no influence over our ageing.

SUMMARY
This section has demonstrated how important our thoughts and feelings are to our health and wellbeing in later life. Positive beliefs about our own ageing and positive approaches to dealing with life's challenges are clearly very important. The next section sets out a whole range of ways to cultivate them and put them into practice.

Ageing is not just a physiological process but also a psychological, intellectual, social and cultural process. Our bodies change but at the same time we mature. Ageing is therefore less about the old and more about the new.

Anne Karpf [28]

TEN STEPS
TO AGEING
POSITIVELY©

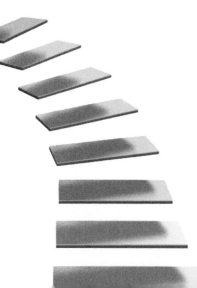

The way you think about ageing and how you view your life in general is vital to your health and wellbeing. A great deal of evidence from scientific research supports this: being positive about yourself is good for you, but being negative is not. This section provides 10 practical steps – a toolkit of exercises for you to use again and again – if you wish to develop a more positive approach to later life.

You are about to embark on a very interesting journey! We suggest that you take some time, possibly 2hrs a week, to take it step by step. You might want to start up a special journal and take notes as you go along. And be aware that some of the exercises are quite challenging and may throw up issues that need some time to work through. So don't rush at it - take your time.

The steps are set out in a logical fashion, but there may be some steps that you might choose to do before others. Whatever order you undertake them we do advise that you look at them all. They hang together as a complete package.

STEP ONE:
SET YOUR INTENTION TO AGE POSITIVELY

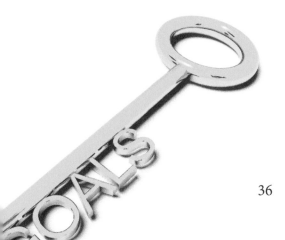

If you want to achieve something in later life you must be clear in your mind about what it is you want to accomplish. In other words, you need to 'set your intention'. You need to think through what 'ageing positively' means to you in order to increase your chances of achieving it.

Comprehensive research involving around 40,000 participants in at least eight countries shows that setting specific mental goals increases performance on more than 100 different tasks – a remarkable fact that provides encouragement for us all!

"People have the power to actively control their lives through purposeful thought; this includes the power to program and reprogram their subconscious, to choose their own goals, to pull out from the subconscious what is relevant to their purpose and to ignore what is not, and to guide their actions based on what they want to accomplish." [29]

SIX KEYS TO SETTING YOUR GOALS

Setting an intention doesn't guarantee that you will achieve what you want, but it does improve your chances greatly. And your chances of success are improved even further if you learn how best to set your goals. There are 6 keys to setting your goals:

• Describe your goals, aims or intentions in **positive** language rather than couching them in negative terms. Thinking about a positive outcome is psychologically much more powerful than avoiding – or fearing – a negative one. For example, 'aiming to achieve a satisfying later life' is much more likely to succeed than 'aiming to avoid loneliness in old age'.

• Make sure your future goals are **realistic** and possible to achieve. There is no point setting yourself unrealistic goals.

• Be as **precise** as possible. For example, aiming to 'have a happy old age' is probably too broad and ill defined. Whereas, aiming 'to achieve the specific goals I have set for the next 5 years' is likely to be much more effective.

• Make a clear **personal commitment** to attaining your goal or intention. Be sure you really want it 'in your heart of hearts'.

• **Compare and contrast** the future you want to achieve with your present situation. Articulate how things are for you now and then be clear about how different you would like your future to be. What will you see, hear of feel differently once you have achieved your goals.

• Look ahead and **predict any hindrances** that might prevent you from achieving your goals and make a plan to overcome them. For example, do you think your family or work commitments might get in the way and distract you? Or do you have a habit of undermining yourself as you attempt to achieve your goals? Whatever it is, be aware of it and think of what actions or plans you could use to tackle it.

Define 'positive ageing' in your own terms, for yourself. Think about it, mull it over and make lots of notes, using the following for guidance:

Describe what you want to achieve in positive terms, i.e. what kind of later life would you prefer to live. Be clear in your own mind that what you are seeking to achieve is within your own control. Remember to avoid using negative terms, but do be clear in your own mind about the sort of old age that you **don't** want to have.

Be as specific and as precise as you can.

Ask yourself questions such as:

■ What exactly is most important to me about ageing positively?

■ How am I going to make it happen?

■ Where and when would I experience it?

■ How would I know that I've achieved my goal?

■ What would positive ageing look and feel like?

When your thoughts are taking shape and crystallising into the kind of goal and intention that you think is worth aiming for, look inside yourself and double check that you want this outcome. Do you really want to age positively in this way? If you could achieve this state of being in the future, would you really want it?

When you're ready, write down your thoughts on good quality paper and in your best handwriting! Such a 'statement' will give your intention more status in your mind.

Now you are ready to make the journey!

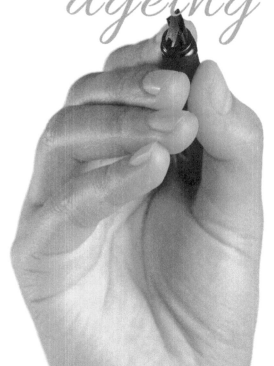

STEP TWO:
FIND OUT WHAT YOU BELIEVE ABOUT YOUR OWN AGEING

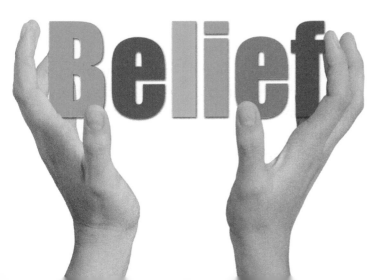

A belief is something that we hold to be true. It guides how we relate to the world we live in and, in a sense, determines how we experience some aspects of life. It comes from personal experience or from the influence of others. A few beliefs are original; many are borrowed.

Mahatma Gandhi summarised very well how influential beliefs can be on our lives:

> *"Your beliefs become your thoughts,*
> *Your thoughts become your words,*
> *Your words become your actions,*
> *Your actions become your habits,*
> *Your habits become your values,*
> *Your values become your destiny."*

SELF-FULFILLING PROPHECIES

To a large extent, our beliefs determine how we experience life. Many beliefs are self-fulfilling prophecies: we believe that something will turn out in a certain way and – surprise, surprise – that is how it turns out. Our beliefs also tend to determine how we interpret what happens to us and, in doing so, confirm the beliefs we had in the first place!

So why is this important? Well, first of all, many of our beliefs are not objectively true. They are not 'facts'; they are interpretations we have made about the world. This is OK as long as our beliefs are helpful. The trouble comes when they are unhelpful – and this is particularly common when it comes to thinking about ageing. Most of our beliefs about ageing are very negative – and if we are not careful, we can set up a lot of self-fulfilling prophecies about how terrible old age is!

DANGERS OF NEGATIVE BELIEFS

We must not underestimate the seriousness of these negative ageist beliefs. Indeed, they can have a life-threatening impact. A piece of ground-breaking research published in 2002 by Becca Levy in America[30] revealed a strong causal link between the negative attitudes that people held towards their own ageing process and their subsequently reduced lifespan. The research showed unequivocally that:-

Those with a negative outlook towards their own ageing died, on average, 7.5 years earlier than other people with a more positive view.

What this means is that negative beliefs about ageing can actually reduce how long we live, even more so than being obese, a smoker, or having high cholesterol or high blood pressure – all of which only shorten life by about 4 years!

The implications of this research are very important and the authors pull no punches in their analysis:

"If a previously unidentified virus was found to diminish life expectancy by over 7 years, considerable effort would probably be devoted to identifying the cause and implementing a remedy. In the present case, one of the likely causes is known: societally sanctioned denigration of the aged."[30]

Ageist stereotypes don't have to be consciously understood or 'visible' to have an impact. The fact is they do have an impact, but how does it work? The self-fulfilling prophecy could well be a factor: if we believe that getting older means that we will inevitably get ill – well then, that is what is very likely to happen. And if people expect they will decline, they may be more likely to interpret some of their experiences in life as evidence of decline. Then their behaviour becomes more 'oldish' than it actually warrants, and so sets a negative spiral in motion.

Negative beliefs can operate in other more medical ways. For example, research has shown that attitudes affect how we respond to stress [30]. So, rather than people seeing stress positively – as part of how life challenges from time to time, people can become overwhelmed by it. This in turn can even go so far as to reduce people's 'will to live'. [30]

TWO KEY MESSAGES
All the research concerning this step provides us with two key messages:

• Firstly, ageism is no joke; it does real damage to people's lives. Negative ideas about age and ageing can shorten life, limit health and reduce our wellbeing in a number of other ways.

• The second message is more positive. If people can replace their negative attitudes towards ageing with more positive ones, then their health, wellbeing and life expectancy could be significantly improved.

This exercise is designed to help you do two things: firstly, to surface what thoughts you have about ageing; and secondly, to assess how helpful or otherwise they are.

Take a few moments to answer the following question:
- What beliefs do you currently hold about your life from now on?
- What exactly do you believe about your own ageing?

Write down your answers.

You might for example believe that you don't have long to live because both of your parents died young. Or you might believe that it is all going to be rather boring because you will gradually loose your health and fitness. Or you might believe that later life is going to be the best part of your life because you don't have to be responsible for anyone else now.

Don't censor yourself or come up with the ideas that you think are 'acceptable'. Allow your mind free rein to think about your own ageing. You might find it helpful to visualise yourself at different ages and in different situation, or try thinking about older people you know or are aware of.

Now look at what you have written and consider the following questions:

- Which of these beliefs are likely to be helpful to you?
- Which of these beliefs could limit your future wellbeing?

There is a way of dealing with death that makes ageing much easier: paradoxically, it's thinking about our own mortality more not less and, incorporating it into our daily lives. Death needs to accompany us through life, and not stalk us... Coming to terms with our mortality isn't easily achieved, or a single event – it's a lifelong process. Accepting death involves a kind of mourning – for oneself. It can also excite anger over the ways in which life has disappointed us, and we've disappointed others... It demands a letting go of one's sense of omnipotence, a facing up to finitude. There's something humbling about it.

Anne Karpf [28]

STEP THREE: REPLACE NEGATIVE OR UNHELPFUL BELIEFS WITH POSITIVE ONES

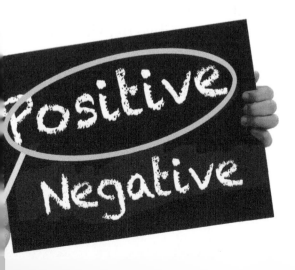

id the previous exercise reveal any beliefs that could be unhelpful to you as you age? Or any beliefs that could limit your future wellbeing? If so, the next step is to replace them with beliefs that are more likely to produce better outcomes for you in later life.

The idea of 'replacing beliefs' can sound strange to many people. Beliefs are often thought of as 'truths' and therefore cannot simply be replaced or changed. But when you think about it a little you can begin to see that most beliefs are partial representations of reality – they are not reality themselves. There are usually 'two sides to a story' and you have a choice about which you want to believe.

This is particularly true when looking into the future. No-one can really know what is going to happen, so whatever beliefs we have about the future are not 'true' or 'real' – they are choices about what we think will happen based on our view of the world.

In Step Two we saw how beliefs tend to act as self-fulfilling prophecies. But self-fulfilling prophecies are not negative by definition. They can be positive, too. Now you have to use this to your advantage: instead of letting negative beliefs about ageing predominate in your life, you need to accentuate some positive ideas about how you are going to grow old. And so you nurture positive beliefs that become positive self-fulfilling prophecies. And the more you nurture them, the more you develop a positive vision of later life – and then there is a much greater chance that things will turn out the way you want them to.

What follows is a powerful step-by-step process for replacing negative, limiting or unhelpful beliefs about your later life with more positive, helpful ones.

This 13-step exercise comes from the field of Neuro Linguistic Programming and is very effective in changing beliefs about the future [31]. It is a challenging exercise. It is best undertaken as part of a group exercise, but it is nevertheless very possible to do on your own.

Find a quiet and private space in which to undertake this exercise. Sit in a comfortable chair and use a notebook if you need to.

1. Firstly, from the previous exercise, identify a belief about your own ageing process that is unhelpful.
2. Next, identify a belief that would be more useful, i.e. a more positive belief about your future
3. Imagine a space on the floor in front of you. This is for the unhelpful belief. Physically step into this space and state the unhelpful belief – either in your head or out loud. Then step out of that space.
4. Imagine a different space on the floor in front of you. This is for your new, more helpful belief.
5. Staying where you are, ask yourself "When I hold this new belief what will I notice that is different? As I practice holding this new belief, how will I experience it? What will I see, hear and feel? What are the benefits?"
6. Now step into the space for the new belief and state all the benefits in the present tense as if they were

already true. Experience in that space what it is like to hold the new belief.

7. Now ask yourself: "Does anything about the belief need changing for it to be congruent with every part of me"? In other words, does it feel completely comfortable or are there some elements of the belief that don't feel quite right? Is there something about the new belief that doesn't quite ring true for you?

8. Step out of the space of the new belief.

9. If any parts of the belief didn't feel quite right consider what changes, if any, you need to make. Then repeat steps 5, 6, 7 and 8 until the new belief feels solid.

10. Step back into the space of the new belief. Ask yourself: "Will I now adopt and live by this belief and enjoy its benefits?" Think about all the benefits of the new belief in the future.

11. Step out of the space, holding onto the new belief in your mind, and step into the space of the old belief. Ask yourself: "What has happened to the old belief?"

12. If the new belief now fits well, the old belief will be redundant and you will find it difficult to feel that it has any power. You are now finished with it. Step out of the space of the old belief.

13. If the old belief resurfaces at any time in your mind, repeat the process from step 2.

If you had more than one unhelpful or negative belief about ageing then you would undertake this process for each of them.

STEP FOUR:
CREATE A POSITIVE MENTAL IMAGE OF YOURSELF AS AN OLDER PERSON

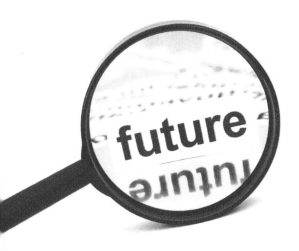

W ith your mind fresh from establishing helpful beliefs about ageing, it is now important to create a strong, positive and attractive mental image of yourself as an older person.

One very useful technique that can help you is visualisation. This is simply a form of 'mental rehearsal'. You create images in your mind of having or doing whatever it is you want. You repeat these images over and over again. Research shows this technique is extremely effective in producing a desired outcome.

The evidence suggests that your mind plays an important role in creating your experience. It may therefore be possible to 'programme' your mind and body to act in a certain way to gain positive results. It has been found that mental practices can enhance motivation, increase confidence and self-efficacy, improve performance of physical tasks and prime your brain for success.

THE POWER OF VISUALISATION

Visualisation is a crucial technique in the world of sport. Seasoned athletes use vivid, highly detailed internal images and run-throughs of their entire performance, engaging all their senses in their mental rehearsal. Two golfers swear by it: Tiger Woods has used visualisation since his pre-teen years and Jack Nicklaus has said that:

"I never hit a shot, not even in practice, without having a very sharp in-focus picture of it in my head".

Russian scientists showed that Olympic athletes who received 50% mental training with 50% physical training produced better performance results than those who received less mental training or none at all. This indicates that certain types of mental training, such as consciously rehearsing specific mental states, can have significant measurable effects on biological performance.

Visualisation can be effective in other fields, too. For example, musicians find it enhances their performance [32] and medical students use it to learn surgical skills [33]. It is also proving valuable in the rehabilitation of patients with motor disturbances following lesions of the central nervous system [34]. By activating certain brain structures selectively it seems to improve the subsequent control and execution of physical movements.

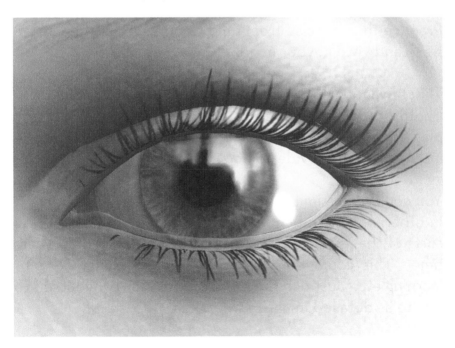

EXERCISE: VISUALISING YOUR FUTURE IMAGE

In the context of looking at our later lives visualisation is a very important technique. We are constantly surrounded by very negative images of older people and they seep into our consciousness. We need to take some concrete steps to counter this.

Find a quiet and private place. Take some time to visualise how you would like to look in 20 years. Try and create as rich and detailed an image as possible.

To help you, think of an older person you know (or from the media) who you find attractive or positive in some way. What is it about them that you find most positive? To what extent do you have some of their characteristics?

Practice this exercise from time to time to keep the image fresh and vivid in your mind.

Those wanting to be particularly adventurous could use Photoshop or other digital photography tools to create and play around with their image! There are resources on the internet which provide some guidance on how to do this

You could do a similar exercise which focuses on 'activity'. In other words, you could take some time to visualise the sorts of things that you would like to be doing in 20 years time. This could be about work or leisure activities or learning etc. Just use the same process - allow yourself to create as detailed images as possible.

STEP FIVE:
MAXIMISE YOUR OPTIMISTIC OUTLOOK

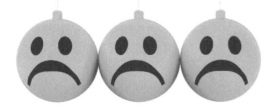

An optimistic outlook on life is good for you. The evidence is overwhelming: it improves longevity, physical health and emotional wellbeing. Optimism is therefore an essential ability to cultivate. And yes, it can be learned! Consciously generating an optimistic framework towards getting older is important for us all, even if we tend to be generally optimistic in other areas of life.

WHAT IS OPTIMISM?

Many think of optimism as a sort of 'happy-clappy, everything is great' approach to life. Others think optimism is unrealistic and fails to understand or acknowledge the difficulties in life. However, a true approach to optimism is nothing like either of these.

Let's think of optimism as one habitual way to interpret what happens to us in life. Martin Seligman, an American psychologist who has written and researched extensively on this subject, explains that there are three dimensions to how people think about a difficult situation that happens to them:

• Is the situation going to last forever or will it pass quite quickly? **Permanence**

• Does it affect many areas of my life or just the one that it first impacted on? **Pervasiveness**

• To what extent do I have control over the situation? **Personalisation**

Martin Seligman's research has shown that, with reference to these three dimensions, optimists and pessimists react to difficult situations in life in very different ways:

- **Optimistic** people tend to interpret their troubles as: transient; are specific to the one situation they relate to; and are things that they have some control over.

- **Pessimistic** people tend to believe that their troubles: last forever; undermine everything they do; and are something that they have little or no control over.

If you think you're more of a pessimist than an optimist, don't despair. Optimism can be learned! But before you start this, try the **Optimism Test** on the website *Authentic Happiness* **(www.authentichappiness.sas.upenn.edu/testcenter)** to discover just how optimistic or pessimistic you are and therefore how much effort you will need to put into the following exercise – cultivating optimism.

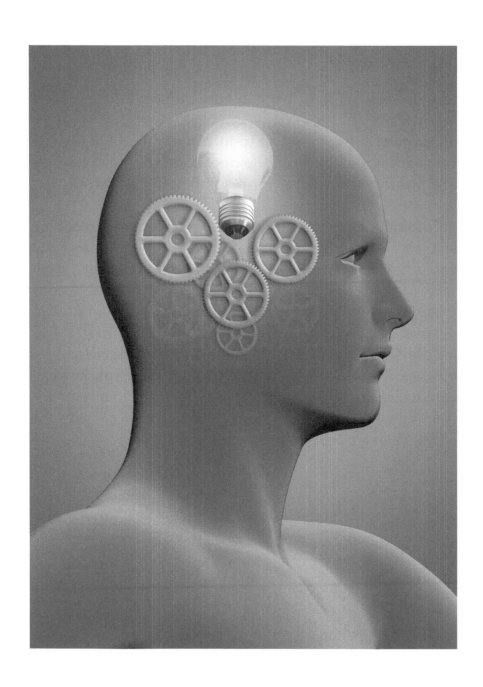

Martin Seligman has developed what he calls the **'ABCDE strategy'** as a way of increasing a person's optimism. In essence, it involves recognising and then disputing pessimistic thoughts.

The key to disputing your pessimistic thoughts is to first recognise them and then to treat them as if they were uttered by another person – someone who might be very happy to see you miserable!

The **ABCDE strategy** works like this:

ADVERSITY This is the incident or trigger associated with a pessimistic thought. What is it that started you to think in this negative way?

BELIEFS What is the thought that you automatically have when this incident or trigger occurs? For example, you might see an older person in a wheelchair and find yourself automatically thinking *"That will be me when I get older – how horrible!"*.

CONSEQUENCES What are the usual consequences of the thought? In the example above, the usual consequences might be that you feel worried and anxious at the thought of getting older.

DISPUTATION This is the crucial step. This is where you begin to dispute or argue against your negative thought. There are a number of ways of making disputations convincing:

Evidence: show that your negative thought is factually incorrect. In the example above, many older people don't get physical impairments, and even if they do, the overwhelming majority of them still rate their health and wellbeing as good or very good.

Implications: even if the thought is true, assess the implications and de-catastophise. In other words, we tend to 'think the worst' when something negative happens. In reality, the worst seldom if ever happens - so we need to remember that and keep our worries and fears in context. So, in the example above, even if I do end up in a wheelchair, I may actually be OK about it and even enjoy the attention sometimes.

Usefulness: sometimes the consequences of holding a belief matter more than its truth. In other words, it is sometimes worth challenging some beliefs just on the grounds that they are so destructive and unproductive, and that it is best to move on from them, even though they might contain a grain of potential truth. In the example above, I might well end up in a wheelchair and I might hate it, but what is the point in thinking about that now at this stage in my life – it might never happen.

ENERGISATION This is what you feel when you successfully dispute your belief. You feel better!

We recommend that you consciously use this **ABCDE strategy** for a number of weeks as you think about your ageing process. And keep a record of your negative or pessimistic thoughts and the ways you disputed them.

STEP SIX:
INCREASE YOUR SENSE OF GRATITUDE

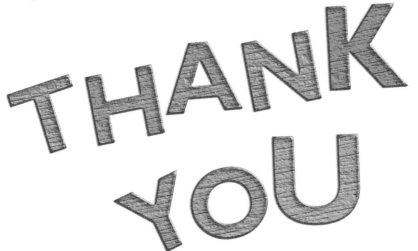

Being thankful for what we have now – or have experienced in the past – can provide a very powerful boost to our health and wellbeing. This is particularly important as we age and become more likely to experience loss. Loss has the potential to make us bitter and resentful. On the other hand, gratitude for what we still have can be a powerful antidote.

Research has shown that the more that we think back upon pleasant experiences, the more we are able to enjoy our lives. Happiness stems from our thoughts; positive thoughts (such as memories of things we are grateful for) produce positive health and wellbeing.

Many studies [35] show that people who regularly keep a gratitude journal report fewer illness symptoms, feel better about themselves and are more optimistic about the future. The research is clear: grateful people are happier, less depressed, less stressed and more satisfied with their lives.

EXERCISE: CULTIVATING GRATITUDE

Start by taking the **Gratitude Survey** on the Authentic Happiness website **(www.authentichappiness.sas.upenn. edu:testcenter)**

Completing this test will give you a ranking of your natural propensity to gratitude. If you score low on this scale you might want to spend a bit more time on this exercise.

Cultivating gratitude is all about getting into a regular way of thinking and remembering. Try the following approach.

Think back over the previous 24 hours and write (on separate lines) up to five things - events, occurrences, kindnesses, coincidences, etc - that you could genuinely be grateful or thankful for. Keep this in a special journal and repeat daily.

And try to increase the impact of gratitude by conjuring up an image in your mind of the positive situation or event. This works because, by remembering specific situations, we are actually recreating the experience in our minds. So a positive memory produces an experience that is almost as good as the real thing.

Do this once a week for several weeks. As time goes by, can you notice a difference in your sense of gratitude and awareness of the good things in your life?

Among the other states that need to be cultivated in preparation for old age, as well as during it, are mourning and gratitude. Old age, says Erikson, is a time of relinquishing - friends, old roles, even possessions that belonged to earlier stages of life. Yet at every stage of life some attachments need to be given up for others to develop, in order to move forward. Such losses and endings are a kind of bereavement and are bound to recur throughout our lives, especially at periods of greatest transition. We need to acknowledge and mourn them if they're not to impede change. This is one of the 'developmental tasks' of ageing, at every age.

Anne Karpf [28]

STEP SEVEN:
BE MINDFUL AND EXPERIENCE THE PRESENT MOMENT

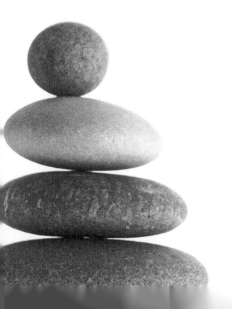

Mindfulness is a very powerful capability for improving your health and general wellbeing in later life. You learn to notice what is occurring in your present moment experience, with an attitude of openness and non-judgmental acceptance.

"Mindfulness is paying attention in a particular way, on purpose, in the present moment, and non-judgmentally." [36]

The research evidence for the benefits of mindfulness is impressive and growing. The following are some of the key areas in which mindfulness can bring powerful results:

PHYSICAL HEALTH

Many clinical trials reveal the significantly positive impact meditation can have on physical health[37]. For example, one long-term randomised trial[38] evaluated the impact of meditation on the death rates of over 200 men and women, average age 71, who had mildly elevated blood pressure. The subjects participated in a meditation programme and were tracked for up to 18 years. The results showed that the meditation programme reduced death rates by 23%. Further analysis showed a 30% decrease in the rate of cardiovascular mortality and a 49% decrease in the rate of mortality due to cancer in the meditation group compared with control group.

MENTAL HEALTH

Mindfulness has also been shown to significantly reduce the chances of suffering depression. It also reduces the likelihood of relapse by about 40–50% in people who have suffered three or more previous episodes of depression [39]. The National Institute for Health and Care Excellence (NICE) has now recommended Mindfulness Based Cognitive Behavioural Therapy for those with a history of three or more episodes in their guidelines for the management of depression.

EMOTIONAL WELLBEING AND RESILIENCE

Mindfulness meditation can improve our ability to deal with all the challenges that life can throw up. It increases our resilience by improving our early detection of stress-causing situations and thereby increases our ability to cope with them effectively [39]. It also reduces our tendency to obsessively 'ruminate', thereby reducing the sort of thought processes that can play a role in producing stress and mental health problems. It improves our awareness of subtle emotional feelings that are so important to the regulation of our emotions [40].

ANTI-AGEING EFFECT

Some research suggests that meditation may provide protection against physical ageing. For example, meditation has been shown to extend the length of 'telomeres', which are the 'cellular markers of ageing'. They are protective structures that cap the ends of chromosomes, the compressed DNA material inside the nucleus of human cells and mitochondria.

Telomeres are necessary for a cell to divide in a healthy way, but each time a normal cell divides, the telomeres become shorter and shorter. Ultimately, the cell's telomeres become so short that they can no longer divide, with the result that the cell dies. Telomere length is therefore an indicator of the ageing of each cell. Many common diseases of ageing are associated with shorter telomeres: cancer, diabetes, osteoarthritis, osteoporosis and cardiovascular disease.

Research shows that meditation practice lengthens telomeres. So it may be possible that regular mindfulness meditation practice may consequently slow the rate of cellular ageing.

"We have found that meditation promotes positive psychological changes, and that meditators showing the greatest improvement on various psychological measures had the highest levels of [the chromosome protecting enzyme] telomerase."
Clfford Saron, University of California, Davis Center for Mind and Brain.

Other work points towards the potential for meditation to give another kind of protection against ageing. Research [41] has established that regular meditation practice may slow age-related thinning of certain parts of the brain. In other words, the study, certain parts of the brains of 40 to 50-year-old meditators (parts which are known to get thinner with age) were similar in average thickness to those of 20 to 30-year-old meditators and controls. The incidence of physical changes in the brain is beginning to be more widely researched and is now commonly referred to as 'neuro plasticity'.

COPING WITH CHRONIC PAIN
Many hospital pain clinics now prescribe mindfulness meditation to help patients cope with the suffering arising

from a wide range of diseases. The research evidence is very strong. Mindfulness can dramatically reduce pain and the emotional reaction to it, with some trials suggesting that pain 'unpleasantness' levels can be reduced by 57% [42]. Clinical trials show that mindfulness improves mood and quality of life in chronic pain conditions such as fibromyalgia and lower back pain [43], in chronic functional disorders such as irritable bowel syndrome and in challenging medical illnesses such as multiple sclerosis and cancer.

RELISHING LIVED EXPERIENCE
As we get older there is no doubt that time appears to speed up. Months fly past in what seem like a matter of days. We can find ourselves rushing headlong towards the finish line – death! Wouldn't it be better if we could notice and savour our moment-to-moment lived experience? Or as Professor Mark Williams from Oxford University and co-developer of Mindfulness Based Cognitive Therapy puts it *"Wouldn't you rather live your life than live in your head? If you were truly alive to your current experience, rather than day-dreaming it away in endless thoughts, you could effectively double your life expectancy!"*

In an interview with the television dramatist Dennis Potter, weeks before his death in 1994, he talked eloquently about experiencing and savouring the present moment. He talked about the plum blossom in his garden.

"Last week, looking at it through the window as I'm writing, I see it is the whitest, frothiest, blossomest blossom that ever could be... The nowness of everything is absolutely wondrous, and if only people could see that... there's no way of telling you,

70

you have to experience the glory of it. The fact is, if you see the present tense, boy, do you see it! And boy, can you celebrate it!"

For Potter it was his impending death that allowed him to "see the present tense" and witness the "blossomest blossom". That awareness of death is not, however, the only way to achieve this intensity of lived experience. Mindfulness meditation is an effective way of improving people's ability to pay attention to present moment experiences and experience them with a similar intensity.

This short breathing space meditation is a great introduction to mindfulness practice. In fact it compresses the core elements of mindfulness into three steps of roughly one minute each. It is the sort of thing you can factor into a regular time in your day or use at those times when you get particularly stressed.

STEP 1:
BECOMING AWARE

Sit comfortably in an erect posture. If possible, close your eyes. Then, bring your awareness to your inner experience and acknowledge it, asking: what is my experience right now?

■ What thoughts are going through your mind? As best you can, acknowledge thoughts as mental events.

■ What feelings are here? Turn towards any sense of discomfort or unpleasant feelings, acknowledging them without trying to make them different from how you find them.

■ What body sensations are here right now? Perhaps quickly scan the body to pick up any sensations of tightness or bracing, acknowledging the sensations, but, once again, not trying to change them in any way.

STEP 2:
GATHERING AND FOCUSING ATTENTION

Now, redirecting the attention to a narrow 'spotlight', move in close to the physical sensations of the breath in the abdomen... expanding as the breath comes in... and falling back as the breath goes out. Follow the breath all the way in and all the way out. Use each breath as an opportunity to anchor yourself into the present. And if the mind wanders, gently escort the attention back to the breath.

STEP 3:
EXPANDING ATTENTION

Now, expand the field of awareness around the breathing so that it includes a sense of the body as a whole, your posture and facial expression, as if the whole body was breathing. If you become aware of any sensations of discomfort or tension, feel free to bring your focus of attention right in to the intensity by imagining that the breath could move into and around the sensations. In this way you are helping to explore the sensations, befriending them, rather than trying to change them in any way. If they stop pulling for your attention, return to sitting, aware of your whole body, moment by moment.

THE HOURGLASS SHAPE OF THE BREATHING SPACE

Try viewing your awareness during the **Breathing Space** as forming the shape of an hourglass. The wide opening at the top of an hourglass is like the **first step** of the Breathing Space. In this, you open your attention and gently acknowledge whatever is entering and leaving awareness.
The **second step** of the Breathing Space is like the narrowing of the hourglass's

73

neck. It's where you focus your attention on the breath in the lower abdomen. You focus on the physical sensations of breathing, gently coaxing the mind back to the breath when it wanders away. This helps to anchor the mind - grounding you back in the present moment.

The **third step** of the Breathing Space is like the broadening base of an hourglass. In this, you open your awareness. In this opening, you are opening to life as it is, preparing yourself for the next moments of your day. Here you are, gently but firmly, reaffirming a sense that you have a place in the world - your whole mind–body, just as it is, in all its peace, dignity and completeness.

LEARNING MORE

Those who do want to cultivate this skill and learn more about mindfulness are advised to:

■ Book onto a **Mindfulness Based Stress Reduction (MBSR)** course. A quick search on the internet will find one available in most communities. It is a structured 8-week course that has been proven to have many health benefits.

■ Search the internet for an online meditation guide - there are hundreds of sites, but you might want to start with this one **www.bemindful.co.uk**

■ Read about mindfulness in a book. Three books particularly recommended are:

● For a purely secular and psychological focussed approach *Mindfulness: a practical guide to finding peace in a frantic world,* **Mark Williams and Danny Penman, Piatkus Books, 2011**

- For a secular Buddhist approach *Life with full attention: a practical course in mindfulness,* **Maitreyabandhu, Windhorse Publications, 2009**

- For those with an illness or chronic pain *Mindfulness for Health: a practical guide to relieving pain, reducing stress and restoring wellbeing,* **Vidyamala Burch and Danny Penman, Piatikus, 2013**

STEP EIGHT:
REVIEW YOUR LIFE

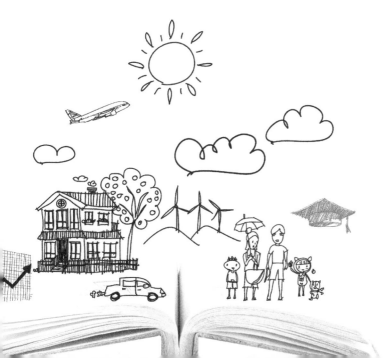

A s we go through life we gather a lot of experience and personal insights. There comes a time when it is useful to look back at all that experience and 'take stock'. Some people refer to this as undertaking a **'life review'**.

"Experience doesn't make people wise. It is reflection on experience that makes us wise"[44]

A life review involves the recalling and re-experiencing of life events. This can help us to accept negative events in the past, resolve past conflicts and find meaning and worth in life. A number of psychologists see this as an essential process for our mental health and wellbeing in later life.

Some might think of a life review as 'wallowing in the past' and argue that it is unhelpful and backward-looking. However, the research suggests otherwise. In one study [45], researchers found that people who seemed to have done the most reflection on their past also exhibited the greatest amount of interest in their future. So, paradoxically, remembering the past can be a very powerful aid to creating the sort of future we want.

A life-review can also be a way of re-interpreting our past in a way which is much more helpful to our present. It may help us to 'become what we might have been'. Jane Fonda, a popular exponent of the life review, suggests that we can go back over our earlier lives and work to change our relationships to the people and the events in our past. She talks about doing a life review *"to poultice the wounds of youth with the forgiveness of age"* [46]. There is a sense here of revising and changing how we feel about past events.

In general, the research indicates a number of wide-ranging benefits:

- reduced levels of stress, anxiety and sense of failure [47]

- improved ability to cope with ageing and death [48]

- decreased levels of depression [49]

- increased psychological wellbeing [50]

- increased life satisfaction and self-esteem [51]

- increased ability to cope and deal with new situations effectively [52]

- less obsessive rumination, and instead a greater sense of wellbeing [53]

The final stage, Erikson maintained, offers us the opportunity to establish an integrated self, to draw on the sustenance of the past (memories, experiences, and achievements) while still retaining a vital involvement in the present. It gives us the chance to see our life as a whole, to come to terms with its meaning, purpose and shape, instead of thinking of it as a series of discrete atomised stages. There is an important reason for reconceiving our life in this way before we reach old age. Connecting with our future self allows us to develop earlier the resources that will serve us better later - resources like the ability to make new friends when we lose old ones, to accept help graciously, to value internal resources as much as external ones, and to be able to let go.

Anne Karpf [28]

There are a number of ways of approaching a life review. Here are three options:

OPTION 1: ASK FOR GUIDANCE

Find a skilled helper who is experienced in active listening or counselling. Having someone else to guide you through the process can be particularly helpful for those people who have major conflicts, regrets or unresolved issues in their past. Many psychologists agree that a conscious and guided process is indeed very helpful, particularly as a way of dealing with possible regrets and feelings of failure.

OPTION 2: DO IT YOURSELF

Undertake the process yourself. This is a particularly good option if you generally feel quite positive about your past. Start out by:

■ Collecting together physical items from the past that have been important to you or are connected with an important event in your life.
■ Visiting places you have enjoyed or places that have had a particular meaning in the past
■ Searching out old photographs and family albums, scrapbooks or other artefacts
■ Attending school reunions or use the internet to find and connect with people from the past
■ Searching out and listening to music that was important to you when you were younger

■ Interviewing key people from your earlier years. There are a number of 'top tips' for interviewing people, particularly if they are friends or relatives.

● Before you begin be clear about your own goals. Are you interested in the person's whole life or just part of it? If negative material comes up, how will you deal with it? Will the material be made available to others or kept private?

● Interview the person in a quiet room, away from other people, ringing phones, etc.

● Use a good tape recorder instead of taking notes.

● Listen attentively and let the person talk and give them time to access their memories.

● Show respect for the person's integrity and choices even though you may disagree with what they are saying. Save your opinions for later.

● If a person's account of an event differs significantly from the historical record, gently tell them and ask whether that is how they remember it. Often, people genuinely don't remember the exact sequence of events.

● If a person refuses to talk about a particular subject respect their wishes. Reassure them that you won't force them to say anything and offer to skip the whole subject and stick to areas they feel more comfortable talking about. As they relax they may be willing to reveal more on the subject.

Try to organise all the information, memories, etc. into some main areas of your life, such as:

■ Family
■ Friendships

- Loves
- Losses
- Achievements
- Disappointments
- Adjustments to life's changes

You will need to review your memories and ask yourself a number of questions such as:

- What memories do I have of when I was very little?
- What was scary when I was younger?
- How did I feel on my first day at school and how did the other children make me feel?
- Have I done anything that I am ashamed of or don't like to think about?
- Were there any special adults in my younger years who made me feel special?
- Was there anyone who made me feel bad about myself or proud of myself?

STAGES AND TRANSITIONS

For more intensive work try to identify the key developmental stages in your life, such as adolescence, or key transitions in life, such as leaving home, getting married, having children, moving house, divorce, etc. These are likely to be some of the 'developmentally charged' times and therefore provide some of the richest material for your review.

You might want to use a 'life line' (opposite) on which to plot some of the key times and events.

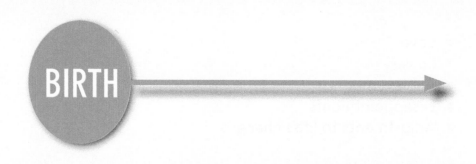

BIRTH

As you review your life line, look for patterns and themes. What have been your strengths, gifts, talents or skills? What do you think your life has been about?

When doing this sort of exercise you should really try to get back to and savour the feelings and mental images associated with them. Try and re-live them vividly. Indeed, actually writing your thoughts out, either in longhand or on the computer, is much more powerful than just 'thinking about' them.

TRANSFORMATIVE POWER OF FORGIVENESS

For many of us there will be some people in our past lives who have hurt us and caused us pain and suffering. Although tempting, it is best not to avoid them. Indeed, much of the value of undertaking a life review is to achieve some sort of resolution to these issues. Martin Seligman provides some very helpful guidance on the transformative power of forgiveness[54]. He advocates the following forgiveness strategy:-

■ **R:** recall the hurt in as objective a way as possible. Do not think of the other person as 'evil'; do not wallow in self pity. Visualize the event and breathe deeply and slowly

■ **E:** empathize – try to understand from the perpetrator's point of view why they hurt you. This is not easy. Make up a plausible story that the perpetrator might say if challenged. To help you do this, remember the following:-

● When others feel their survival is threatened, they will hurt innocents. People who attack others are themselves usually in a state of fear, worry, and hurt
● The situation that a person finds themselves in, and not their underlying personality, can lead to hurting
● People often don't think when they hurt others; they just lash out

■ **A:** the altruistic gift of forgiveness. Recall a time that you have transgressed, felt guilty and were forgiven. This was a gift you were given by another person. Tell yourself that you can rise above hurt and vengeance. If you give the gift grudgingly it will not set you free.

■ **C:** commit yourself to forgive publicly

■ **H:** hold onto the forgiveness. Don't dwell vengefully on the memories, and don't wallow in them. Remind yourself as regularly as necessary that you have forgiven.

Although it is not easy, it can be transformative to imagine the pain that those people who have hurt you probably experienced in their own lives; in particular, the self-hatred that may have led them to hurt you. Trying to feel forgiveness towards them can be very powerful. And commit to never doing these same hurtful things to others or to yourself.

Forgiveness is not erasure or suppression – it is a change of the feeling associations that the memory carries [54]

A life review can take a long time, so enjoy it! And make plenty of notes of your thoughts as you explore your past. As Jane Fonda says:

"Don't edit; just let the ideas flow. Turn them around slowly, in the light, and try to see past the surfaces." [46]

OPTION 3: WRITE YOUR MEMOIRS

A life review can take the form of a memoir or autobiography. You could instead join a writing group and use some of the time to review and write about your earlier life. You can address many of the life areas outlined above. Just the act of writing in a thoughtful way about the past can be transforming.

STEP NINE:
ESTABLISH WHAT IS MOST IMPORTANT TO YOU

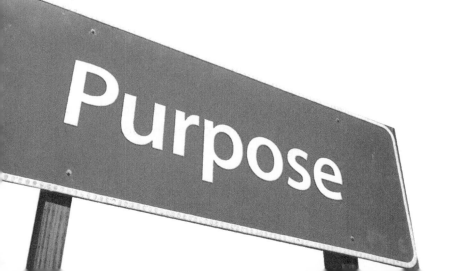

A sense of purpose is one of the most beneficial things for our health and wellbeing in later life. People who know what their life purpose is – 'who know why they wake up in the morning' – live longer, better lives. This is corroborated by the fact that people who tend to live exceptionally long lives – for example, on the Japanese island of Okinawa or in the part of Costa Rica called Nicoya – belong to communities that promote a very strong concept of a sense of purpose. Okinawans call it *ikigai* and Nicoyans call it *plan de vida*.

There is also strong scientific evidence. A large-scale, 11-year study [55] followed healthy people between the ages of 65 and 92, and showed that those who expressed clear goals or purpose lived longer and lived better than those who did not. It also identified that a strong sense of purpose appears to lower the risk of developing dementia by an incredible 2.4 times.

MEANING IN YOUR LIFE

A sense of purpose is very closely aligned to the 'meaning' we attach to our lives. This was very starkly outlined by Viktor Frankl, a prominent Jewish psychiatrist and neurologist, in a book about his experiences in the concentration camps. He concluded that the difference between those who had lived and those who had died came down to one thing: *Meaning*. As far as he could see, those people in the camps who found meaning even in the most horrendous circumstances were far more resilient to suffering than those who did not.

A sense of purpose or meaning in life is obviously a very individual thing and is different for different people. Some of the most common are:

- To make a positive contribution to the rest of society

- To maximise one's potential and personal development

- To be artistically or intellectually creative

- To develop spiritually

- To seek pleasure

BENEFITS OF VOLUNTEERING

For many people, volunteering is a very practical expression of their sense of purpose in life. All the evidence shows that there are significant positive benefits for older people who volunteer. For example, a recent UK study [56] involving over 5,000 older people was able to conclude *"there is strong evidence supportive of a causal interpretation of the relationship between volunteering and wellbeing in later life."*

This investigation of volunteering and older people looked at a number of indicators of wellbeing – depression, quality of life, life satisfaction, and social isolation – and how these were affected by people's involvement in volunteering over a two-year period. A number of key points are worth noting:

- The wellbeing of older volunteers was greater than that of non-volunteers

- The strength of the wellbeing effect increased with the volume of volunteering undertaken, i.e. there is a 'dose effect'

• The relationship between volunteering and wellbeing was not present in those people who stopped volunteering

• Improvement in wellbeing was only present where people felt appreciated for the efforts they put into volunteering.

What is particularly impressive about the high levels of satisfaction is that, in some studies, over half of the volunteers report long-term health difficulties – e.g. arthritis, mobility and heart problems. These kinds of health conditions do not necessarily stop people from actively engaging in their communities.

The following exercise will help you to establish your sense of purpose or what is important to you in life. The basic idea is that, by mentally stepping into your future, you can discover what is important to you now. This then helps you to:

■ See your future from a different perspective

■ Gain some insight into that future

■ Be better informed about the choices and actions you might want to take now in order to improve your chances of getting the future you want.

First, imagine a line on the ground in front of you.

Imagine that one end is the start of your life and at the other end is its conclusion.

Using this time line, metaphorically 'step into your future' by walking to the part that represents the end of your life.

Then look back to 'now' (i.e. to where you have just come from). Take some time to think about what you would want to have achieved once you get to this end point. What will you be really glad you did or became? Alternatively, what might you most regret not having done? You could focus in turn on a number of areas of life - eg. family, friends, work, leisure, health, spirituality / philosophy of life etc.

This should begin to articulate what is most important to you in life and help crystallise your sense of purpose in life.

Step out of your 'time line' and jot down what you have learned and see whether you can articulate your 'sense of purpose' in a few sentences.

STEP TEN:
DEVELOP A LIFE PLAN FOR YOUR LATER YEARS

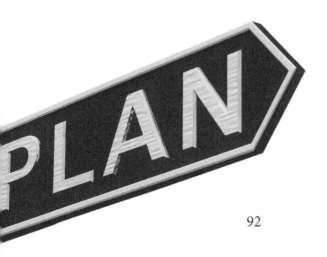

The next and final step is to work out a plan to make your sense of purpose a reality. There are no guarantees here – life is unpredictable – but planning can significantly increase your chances of getting what you want. Jane Fonda argues that *"Luck is opportunity meeting preparation…with preparation and knowledge, with information and reflection, we can try to raise the odds of being lucky, and of making our last three decades the most peaceful, generous, loving, sensual, transcendent time of all: and that planning for it, especially during one's middle years, can help make this so."* [46] It is a bit like "Setting your intention", which we looked at in Step One.

Academic research evidence supports the view that forward planning in life is critical to our health and wellbeing. When there is nothing to look forward to there is little point in living.

This exercise[1] helps you to translate the priorities you uncovered in the previous exercise and turn them into concrete goals.

Firstly, it is important to reflect on how much time we are spending on the different parts of our lives and how satisfied we are with the quality of our lives in each part.

To help you do this try using the image of a pie, with eight slices, each representing an element of your life:-

- work
- family and friends
- learning and self development
- health and fitness
- emotional wellbeing
- leisure and fun
- spiritual / Philosophical life
- civic engagement / volunteering

YOUR CURRENT PIE

The next step is to indicate on your 'current pie':-

- an estimate of the amount of time you currently give to various elements in your life. If you assume 100 hours a week it makes it easier.

[1] Taken from The 3rd Age Life Planning Toolkit, by Margaret Newhouse and Judy Goggin

The following diagram is for illustrative purposes only:

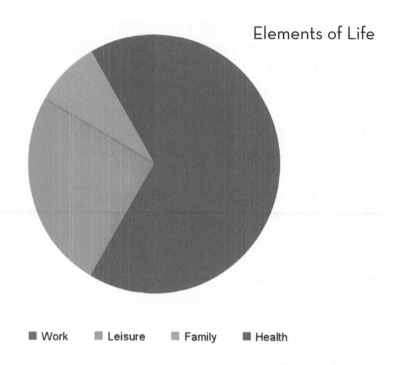

Elements of Life

■ Work   ■ Leisure   ■ Family   ■ Health

■ then give each slice a rating of 1 to 10 based on how satisfied you are with the amount of time you devote to each part in your life right now: **1 = 'the pits'** and **10 = 'fantastic'.**

YOUR FUTURE PIE

Now pick a time 2 to 5 years from now. Draw another pie chart. How would you like the pie to be sliced then? Try to do this quickly and intuitively.

Having reflected on the above exercise, spend some time brainstorming which large-scale goals or outcomes you want to achieve in each of the slices of your 'future pie'.

Write a sentence which encapsulates each.

Be careful how you construct your goals. A successful goal will:

Be specific – broad general statements lack focus and are therefore difficult to achieve

Be realistic – make sure you are not setting yourself up to fail by setting a completely unrealistic outcome

Be positive – set out what you do want to happen, not what you don't want to happen

Be within your control – you can't make others behave the way you want to! So make sure your outcomes are about things that you can make happen

Have evidence of success – think about what signs would let you know whether you have achieved your outcomes.

For each life area write all your outcomes down and be sure to review them periodically. Look at them every three months to keep on top of them and to keep them fresh. It is surprising how the very act of reviewing your goals can help bring them into being. It is the psychological process of keeping them 'live' in your unconscious that makes them begin to come to fruition.

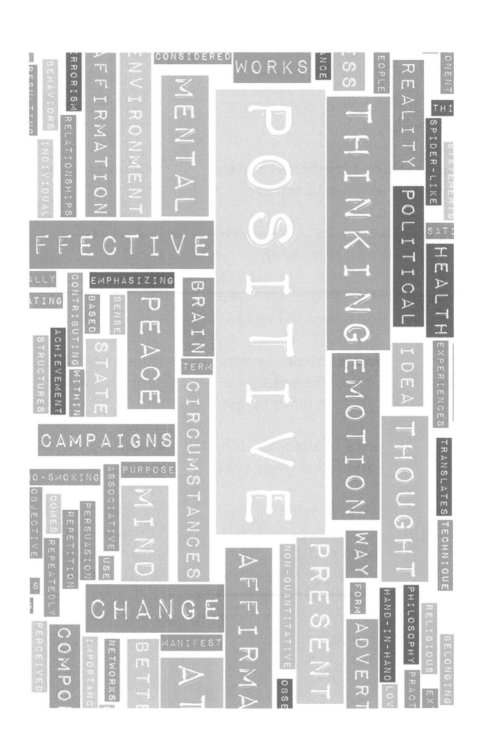

REVIEW

So the journey of personal change in later life has begun! You should now be much better prepared to challenge some of the strong negative attitudes to ageing that are so prevalent in society. We all need to challenge these, particularly the negative thoughts that might tend to re-appear in our own minds.

The more we're able to understand how ageist assumptions shape our thoughts and behaviour, the less hold they will have over us. As we begin to identify the caricatures and prejudices we've internalized and understand their social origins, they become more resistible. And this makes it possible to age more freely – to become more fully ourselves.[28]

Ageing well is not just about exercise and diet. As we have seen in this book, the evidence shows that our thoughts and feelings are incredibly important. What we believe about how our future will turn out can have a big impact on how it actually does. If we go into later life with the idea that - *'it's all down hill'* – then we should not be surprised if it turns out that way. By way of contrast, if we have a positive attitude to ageing, then we are much more likely to have a good experience of later life. Ageing can be actively enriching and be a time of immense growth and satisfaction.

As **Anne Karpf** says in her powerful little book on ageing[28] – *"We can continue to grow as long as we continue to breathe."* We need to challenge the notion that the only good way to age, is not to!

We have learnt that there are many things we can do to actively promote personal change in later life. We can:-

• be clear in our minds about what we want to get out of later life by setting our intentions
• clarify what we truly believe about ageing
• ensure that we replace any negative beliefs with more positive ideas
• develop a vivid mental image of how we want to see ourselves when we are older
• learn to be more optimistic
• be more systematically grateful for what we have in life by concentrating on the positive aspects of our lives
• experience more deeply and savour our time by becoming more mindful
• look back on our lives and gain more insight into who we have been and therefore who we might be in the future
• work out what is most important for us to achieve in the remainder of our lives
• finally, make a plan to ensure that we accomplish the things that we want to.

By successfully undertaking and completing the exercises in this handbook it is possible that we will be able to say that:

"I am motivated by intention, equipped with positive beliefs and powered by a strong mental image of myself, and so brimming with optimism, gratitude and mindfulness, and embracing a clear vision of what's important to me, I embark willingly and open-heartedly on an intriguing life plan that I have mapped out for myself." [2]

[2] Thanks to Pip Morgan

EVALUATION

It is always helpful to reflect on things that we have done or attempted to do in order to increase our learning about ourselves and/or the task we set ourselves. You might therefore want to look back on your experience of undertaking the 10 steps to positive ageing:-

- How did I do?

- What worked well?

- What did I find challenging

FEEDBACK

We are always keen to find out how people experience these ideas and exercises so please feel free to contact us to provide your feedback by emailing **info@positiveageing.org.uk**

CONCLUSION

We hope that the information and exercises contained in this handbook have been useful to you. We believe that, by using the material here, you will be able to take greater control of your ageing process and begin to create the kind of later life that you want. There are no certainties, but we believe that the research evidence is sufficiently strong for us to be confident that following this approach will increase your chances of improving your health and wellbeing in this next phase of your life.

And it has the potential to be a very exciting time. Most of us will spend more time in this phase of later life than we did between being born and finishing at university/college or our apprenticeship! Surely that fact alone warrants spending some quality time, attention and planning on those future years.

Ageing is a process, not a crisis. There has never been a better time to age!

If we can cultivate respect for our own growth and develop the ability to greet our ageing self with both pleasure and realism and without the need to either idealise or deride it's younger incarnation, then we are putting in place important capacities that will serve us our entire lives.

Anne Karpf [28]

REFERENCES

1. de Hennezel, M., *The warmth of the heart prevents the body from rusting: ageing without growing old.* 2011, Australia: Scribe Publications.

2. Rowe, J. and R. Kahn, *Successful Aging.* 1998, New York: Pantheon Books.

3. Bowling, A. and P. Dieppe, *What is successful ageing and who should define it?* BMJ, 2005. 331: p. 1548-1551.

4. Ryff, C.D. and C. Keyes, *The structure of psychological wellbeing revisitied.* Journal of Personality and Social Psychology, 1995. 69: p. 719-727.

5. Deary, I., *Allow for some hard thinking at 85 and over, in Improving later life: understanding the oldest old.* 2013, Age UK: London.

6. Holt-Lunstad, J., T.B. Smith, and J.B. Layton, *Social relationships and mortality risk: a meta-analytic review.* PLoS Med, 2010. 7(7): p. e1000316.

7. Hill, P., *Having a sense of purpose may add years to life.* Psychological Science, 2014.

8. Office for National Statistics, *General Lifestyle Survey.* 2011.

9. Institute for Ageing and Health, *Newcastle 85 plus study.* Newcastle University.

10. Alzheimer's Society, *Dementia 2012: a national challenge.* 2012.

11. Matthews, F.e.a., *A two decade comparison of prevalence of dementia in indfividuals aged 65 and older from three geographical areas in England: results of the Cognitive Function and Ageing Study I and II.* The Lancet, 2013.

12. Office for National Statistics, *Analysis of experimental subjective wellbeing data from the annual population survey.* 2012.

13. Blanchard - Fields F, S.R., Watson T,, *Age differences in emotion regulation strategies in handling everyday problems.* Journals of Gerontology: Psychological Science, 2004. 59: p. 261 - 269.

14. Williams L M, e.a., *The mellow years? Neural basis of improving emotional stability over age.* Journal of Neuroscience, 2006. 26: p. 6422-6430.

15. Carstensen, L., *Evidence for a life span theory of socioemotional selectivity.* Current Directions in Psychological Science, 1995. 4(5): p. 151-156.

16. Deiner, E., *Happy people live longer: Subjective wellbeing contributes to health and longevity.* Journal of Applied Psychology, 2011. 3(1): p. 1-43.

17. Hemingway, H. and M. Marmot, *Psychosocial factors in the aetiology and prognosis of coronary heart disease: systematic review of prospective cohort studies.* British Medical Journal, 1999. 318: p. 1460-1467.

18. Chida, Y. and A. Steptoe, *Positive psychological wellbeing and mortality: a quantitative review of prospective observational studies.* Psychosomatic Medicine, 2008. 70: p. 741-756.

19. Brumett, B., et al., *Prediction of all-cause mortality by the Minnesota Mulitphasic Personality Inventory Optimism-Pessimism Scale scores: Study of a college sample during a 40 year follow up.* Mayo Clinic Proceedings, 2006. 81: p. 1541-1544.

20. Scheier, M., et al., *Dispositional optimism and recovery from coronary artery bypass surgery: the beneficial effects on physical and psychological wellbeing.* Journal of Personality and Social Psychology, 1989. 57(6): p. 1024-1040.

21. Fredman L, H.W.G., Black S, Bertrand RM, Magaziner J,, *Elderly patients with hip fracture with positive affect have better functional recovery over 2 years.* Journal of the

American Geriatrics society, 2006. 54: p. 1074-1081.

22. Kim, E.S., N. Park, and C. Peterson, *Dispositional Optimism Protects Older Adults From Stroke: The Health and Retirement Study.* Stroke, 2011.

23. Giltay, E., F. Zitman, and D. Kromhout, *Dispositional optimism and the risk of depressive symptoms during 15 years follow up: the Zutpen Elderly Study.* Journal of Affective Disorders, 2006. 91(1): p. 45-52.

24. Allison, P., et al., *Dispositional optimism predicts survival status 1 year after diagnosis in head and neck cancer patients.* Journal of Clinical Oncology, 2003. 21(3): p. 543-548.

25. Scheier, M., C. Carver, and M. Bridges, *Optimism, Pessimism and Psychological Well-Being, in Optimism and Pessimism: Implications for Theory, Research and Practice,* E. Chang, Editor. 2001, American Psychological Association: Washington.

26. Kirkwood, T. Newcastle *Initiative on Changing Age: About Ageing.* 2013; Available from: http://www.ncl.ac.uk/changingage/research/ageing/.

27. Carstensen, L., *A long bright future: happiness, health and financial security in an age of increased longevity.* 2009.

28. Karpf, A., *How to age,* ed. T.S.o. Life. 2014, London: Macmillan.

29. Bandura *A, Self-Efficacy: the exercise of control.* 1997, New York: Freeman.

30. Levy, B., et al., *Longevity Increased by Positive Self-Perceptions of Aging.* Journal of Personality and Social Psychology, 2002. 83(2): p. 261-270.

31. O'Connor, J., *NLP Workbook.* 2001, London: Element.

32. Theiller A M, L.L.G., *Effects of mental practice and modelling on guitar and vocal performance.* Journal of General Psychology, 1995. 122(4): p. 329-343.

33. Sanders C W, e.a., *Learning basic surgical skills with mental imagery: using the simulation centre in the mind.* Medical Education, 2008. 42(6): p. 607 - 612.

34. Decety J, I.D.H., *Brain structure participating in mental simulation of motor behaviour: A neuropsychological interpretation.* Acta Psychologica, 1990. 73(1): p. 13-34.

35. Emmons, R., *Thanks!: How the new science of gratitude can make you happier.* 2007: Houghton Mifflin Harcourt.

36. Kabat-Zinn, J., *Full Catastrophe Living.* 1990, United States: Dell Publisher.

37. Grossman, P., et al., *Mindfulness based stress reduction and health benefits: a meta analysis. Journal of Psychosomatic Research,* 2004. 57: p. 35-43.

38. Schneider R, e.a., *Long term effects of stress reduction on mortality of persons over 55 years of age with systemic hypertension.* American Journal of Cardiology, 2005. 95(9): p. 1060-1064.

39. Teasdale, J., et al., *Prevention of relapse/reocurrence in major depression by mindfulness based cognitive therapy.* Journal of Consulting and Clinical Psychology, 2000. 68(615-623).

40. Neilsen L, K.A.W., *Awareness of subtle emotional feelings: a comparison of long term meditators and non meditators.* Emotion, 2006. 6(3): p. 392-405.

41. Lazar, S.W., et al,, *Meditation experience is associated with increased cortical thickness.* Neuroreport, 2005. 16(17): p. 1893-1897.

42. Zeidan F, e.a., *Brain mechanisms supporting the modulation of pain by mindfulness meditation.* Journal of Neuroscience, 2011. 31(14): p. 5540.

43. Morone N E, e.a., *"I felt like a new person" - the effects of mindfulness meditation on older adults with chronic pain: qualitative narrative analysis of diary entries.* Journal of Pain 2008b. 9: p. 841-8.

44. Bateson, M., *Composing a further life: the age of active* *wisdom*. 2010, United States: Random House.

45. Costa P, K.R., *Some aspects of memories and ambitions in centenarians*. Journal of Genetic Psychology, 1967. 110: p. 3-16.

46. Fonda, J., *Prime Time*. 2011, United States: Random House.

47. Gibson, *Owning the past in dementia care: creative engagement with others, in State of the Art in Dementia Care*, M. Marshall, Editor. 1997, Centre for Policy on Ageing.

48. Mosher-Ashley, P.M. and P.W. Barret, *A life worth living: practical strategies for reducing depression in older adults*. Health Professions Press.

49. Watt, L.M. and P. Cappeliez, *Integrative and instrumental reminisence therapies for depression in older adults: Intervention strategies and treatment effectiveness*. Ageing and Mental Health, 2000. 4(2): p. 166-177.

50. Cappeliez, P. and e. al, *Functions of reminisence and emotional regulation among older adults*. Journal of ageing studies, 2008. 22: p. 266-272.

51. Fujiwara, E. and e. al, *Usefulness of reminisence therapy for community mental health*. Pyschiatry and Clinical Neuroscience, 2012. 66(1): p. 74-79.

52. Cappeliez, P. and A. Robitaille, *Coping mediates the relationships between reminisence and psychological wellbeing among older adults*. Ageing and Mental Health, 2010. 14(7): p. 807-818.

53. Torges, C.M., A.J. Stewart, and S. Nolen-Hoeksema, *Regret resolution, ageing and adapting to loss*. Pschology and Ageing, 2008. 23: p. 169-180.

54. Seligman, M., *Authentic Happiness*. 2002, USA: Nicholas Brearley.

55. Butler, K., *Knocking on Heaven's Door: the path to a better way of death*. 2013: Scribner.

56. Nazroo, J. and K. Matthews, *The impact of volunteering on well-being in later life*. 2012, WRVS.

Lightning Source UK Ltd.
Milton Keynes UK
UKOW06f2157110615

253334UK00014B/94/P